D1246079

WHAT REVIEWERS ARE SAYING ABOUT

THEY TOOK MY PROSTATE

CANCER ◊ LOSS ◊ HOPE

"I recommend this book for every man who is contemplating surgery for prostate cancer. For one thing, JP Mac is very funny. I believe his ability to find the absurd and keep his perspective even in the most awkward or discouraging situations is one important reason for his successful recovery. His strong support from his wife, Joy, and their family is another. Finally, he talks about the nitty-gritty aspects of recovering from this life-saving but difficult surgery — something few men are willing to do. He got through it, and got his life back. Reading this might help you get through it, too."

— Janet Farrar Worthington, Co-Author, ***Dr. Patrick Walsh's Guide to Surviving Prostate Cancer***

"Written by perhaps the funniest man I have ever known. A book for the post-New Year's doldrums!"

— Emmy-Award winning writer **Paul Rugg**

THEY TOOK MY PROSTATE

By JP Mac

THEY TOOK MY PROSTATE

CANCER ◊ LOSS ◊ HOPE

By
JP Mac

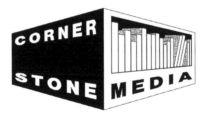

Cornerstone Media
La Cañada, California

ALSO BY JP MAC

Fiction

Hallow Mass
Fifty Shades of Zane Grey
The Little Book of Big Enlightenment

Non-Fiction

Jury Doody

TABLE OF CONTENTS

"Nothing is more dangerous to men than a sudden change in fortune."

— Quintillian

CHAPTER 1

MARK OF THE COBRA

Cringing in discomfort, I stared at the wall, curled up on the examination table like a possum under a shrub. Tissue samples were being harvested from my prostate. Earlier, I'd received a novocaine injection, but the doctor must've bought a bad drum from Amazon because . . . I. felt. everything.

With a noise like a mousetrap closing—*whap!*—the biopsy needle would snag a tissue sample and I would squirm. In addition, a trans-rectal camera had been inserted up my butt like a plumber's snake into a drain.

Operating this trans-rectal camera/biopsy needle was my urologist, Dr. Vaughn Trachmann. Around my age, early 60s, with more salt than pepper in his black hair, he had sad brown eyes, heavy-lidded, sleepy—as if he were perpetually up late. Snipping his tissue samples,

1

Trachmann kept up a distracting patter about an NPR radio program called *A Prairie Home Companion.*

For those who are fuzzy on male anatomy, the prostate is a walnut-sized gland located at the bladder outlet and the junction of the urinary and reproductive tracts. During a routine physical, this is the organ a doctor checks for enlargement when he sticks a finger up a patient's butt. (After which both parties pretend nothing happened.) Situated at a vital biological crossroad, the prostate observes urine and semen exiting a man's body without comment or judgment.

Dr. Trachmann said, "Your prostate appears normal-sized."

"I guess that's good."

Whap!

I squirmed more, said "oww" again, and wriggled like a flat worm on a slide, none of which helped.

Trachmann continued, "I loved that guy who did the sounds for the show. What was his name?"

"I don't know."

Whap!

"Owww, man!"

Prostate gland cells manufacture a protein called prostate specific antigen. (Initially, I wasn't sure what this protein did, suspecting a form of biological busy work.)

An antigen is a toxin that issues an immune response, especially in the production of antibodies. Think of an immune response as a burglar alarm that should be investigated. Had a rodent scuttled past the motion sensor, or was there a thief?

Trachmann said, "Tom Keith, now I remember. He's dead now, but he made some amazing effects."

"How many more samples?"

"Close to the end now."

Whap!

"Shit."

Elevated PSA levels can indicate cancer. During a physical six weeks earlier, a blood test revealed my PSA was borderline high at 4.3, up from 3.2 the previous year. The increase earned me a referral to a urologist. A few weeks later, following a second blood test at Trachmann's office, my PSA jumped again to 6.3. This new level qualified me for the biopsy. And because prostate cancer could be multifocal, meaning multiple tumors might pop up like crabgrass, numerous tissue samples from the prostate periphery were needed to pinpoint any skulking malignancy.

Writhing on the examination table, I hated the whole procedure. When would this miserable biopsy end? Sharp stabbing pains rendered cancer as inconsequential and remote as the icy surface of Europa.

Whap!

I gritted my teeth, "This is really bad."

"Now Butch Thompson, there was a piano player."

Whap!

"Come on."

"Close to the end now."

"You've said that twice."

Whap!

At last Trachmann departed the examination room, carting along a dozen tissue samples. A cute nurse with black horn-rimmed glasses said I could get dressed, leaving me a sheet of post-procedure instructions. Alone in the room, I lay there in my ass-less gown with a throbbing rectal pain. Sliding off the examination table, I glanced back at the white surgical mat, covered in drips and blobs of my blood.

Dazed, I felt like a young actress leaving Harvey Weinstein's hotel room. On a countertop, I spied a roll of paper towels. Tearing off several sheets, I fashioned a "manpon," wedging the papers against my bloody butt, then pulled up my underwear. After dressing, I left the office, realizing I now walked differently.

Outside the medical center, morning traffic zipped along Burbank Boulevard. In a post-biopsy daze, I didn't notice the late July heat. I concentrated on negotiating the sidewalk in my new shuffle. In recalling this unique movement, no comparison springs to mind except that it mitigated rectal pain. Pedestrians passed, aloof, indifferent, this being Los Angeles and home to far weirder things than a funny-walking old guy.

Thank God it was over.

Carefully lowering myself behind the wheel of my car, I hoped this latest medical adventure closed with a negative biopsy. According to my urologist and staunch NPR fan, a man with a PSA level between 4 and 10—6.3 for me—sported a 25% chance that a biopsy would reveal cancer. One in four sucked. Wheeling into traffic, I headed for the freeway, concentrating on what I did best: worrying.

Once, I'd had a career writing TV animation for studios such as Warner Bros. and Disney. But as I grew older, work dried up like California farmland. I'd migrated downstream from well-paid staff jobs, to extensive free-lance work to the occasional mercy script from an old colleague. Alas, my Motion Picture union health care benefits were indexed to how much I worked in a six-month qualifying period.

Lots of script writing equaled lots of qualifying hours, translating into excellent health care benefits for six months. And with my assorted health woes, I'd needed them. Over the last several years I'd undergone three major operations and seemed welded into a loop of discovery-operation-physical therapy-recovery-discovery. However, should I fail to work the necessary hours during a qualifying half-year, my benefits terminated. Then it was off to COBRA town.

COBRA stands for the Consolidated Omnibus Budget Reconciliation Act, a snappy bit of government labeling that meant I could acquire an additional 18 months of union benefits. Of course, I would be required to pay the entire cost of the premium. At that time, the health care premium for my wife Joy and me ran around twelve hundred bucks a month.

Unfortunately, Joy and I were broke.

A Korean grocery truck glided across several lanes, almost hitting a Kia.

Actually, "broke" is the absence of money: we'd plunged into deep Marianas Trench-like debt. As my TV animation star descended, so did Joy's career in magazine production. (CraigsList gobbled up advertising and wiped out numerous publications.) We lowered our overhead, selling a big home and downsizing to a condo. Soon we were burning through our savings and lighting up the credit cards. All our prehistoric appliances made loud, pre-breakdown noises. Joy's auto was a mechanic's ATM, and little frills such as new clothes and vacations fell from our lives like petals from a cherry blossom.

Earlier that year of 2014, two small writing projects at DreamWorks and Warner Bros. brought in some money, but not enough union hours. We were on COBRA vapors, unsure what would happen next. With health care expiring at the end of September, Joy and I spent that spring and summer squeezing in medical and dental exams. As fate decreed, this medical spree resulted in the blood test that discovered my elevated PSA, resulting in the biopsy. Zipping through traffic, I really didn't fancy a new cancer. (I already had one variety.)

Merging onto the 134 freeway, I took a deep breath and relaxed. From the little I'd read, my odds were better than I thought. For one thing, I had no family history of prostate cancer. (We were heart attack people.) For another, a recent physical exam had discovered no cancer symptoms such as an enlarged prostate. For a third, even Trachmann's trans-rectal camera—I think he left the tripod open—recorded my prostate as a normal-sized organ. And fourth, the biopsy carried a 75% chance of returning negative.

A Toyota truck full of lawnmowers cut me off. I honked and smiled.

I'd be fine.

Relieved, I focused on fretting over money.

CHAPTER 2

PROSTATE BEFORE SCIENCE

According to the post-procedure instructions left for me by Cute Nurse, the biopsy might produce interesting after effects. For example, I was apprised that I could urinate blood. (I did.) I was also alerted to the possibility that "you may . . . notice blood or discoloration in your semen if you are sexually active." Really?

Then my wife and I had sex. In the aftermath, there was blood all over my groin, plus blood and semen smeared on the bedding. It looked as if I'd had humped a small animal, then killed it with a hot dog fork. My wife took matters in stride, suggesting I chill. Instead I brooded. Was this mess an omen?

Nine days later I returned to Trachmann's office for my biopsy results. I was ushered into a tiny exam room with a chair, stool, exam table, and counter with a glass jar of cotton balls. On the floor stood a wastebasket with yellow and black Biohazard markings. I read my Kindle and listened to Trachmann consulting other patients through the thin walls.

("Chris Thile is fine, but I really liked the old host.")

A rap on the door: Trachmann with a different cute nurse. This young woman wore teal scrubs and held a laptop. Like a court stenographer, Teal Scrubs typed down everything that was said. (I'm sure it had nothing to do with lawsuits.) No NPR patter for me.

"Your biopsy came back positive."

Numbness.

Trachmann explained my Gleason score, which is a number assessing the aggressiveness of cancer. To better illustrate, he drew diagrams and percentages and cure rates in the margins of my biopsy report. I nodded, uttered sounds, but all I could think was "cancercancercancer." Here's a sample of our dialogue.

Trachmann: "Five of twelve samples tested positive for adenocarcinoma."

Me: "Five, huh?" (*cancercancercancer.*)

Trachmann: ". . . Partin score lets us determine the viability of a surgical cure . . ."

Me: "Uh." (*cancercancercancer.*)

Trachmann: ". . . 38% chance of capsule penetration . . ."

Me: "Oh." (*cancercancercancer.*)

Trachmann: "Read this book by Dr. Patrick Walsh and see me in a week."

Me: "Walsh." (*cancercancercancer.*)

Trachmann: "Make that two weeks. I'm going to Ecuador."

After booking a follow-up appointment with Trachmann's Paperwork Gals, I drifted outside, holding a rolled up copy of my biopsy report like a racetrack program with all the losers circled. I felt sucker-punched. One in four. Well, who needs odds when you've got luck?

In the August sunshine, I shambled to my car, depressed, awash in self-pity, wondering about the future: a 61-year-old guy with cancer, lousy employment prospects, plus no health care in 55 days. I called my wife. With California being a community property state, it was half her disease now. Joy was bummed, but resolute: We'd fight this thing.

Driving home, traffic from the Disney lot flowed onto Buena Vista, slowing my progress to the freeway. Adenocarcinoma? Why me? We lived modestly with lousy appliances, loud drunken neighbors, and no money. Prostate cancer seemed unfair, spiteful, very near to piling on.

After a few days awash in maudlin self-pity, I bought *Dr. Patrick Walsh's Guide to Surviving Prostate Cancer.*

Hefty tome, a mass of material; none of which I would've cared about a week before. Immediately, I learned that treating prostate cancer is tricky because the darn organ is tough to reach. Deep in the pelvis, surrounded as if by ivy-covered walls, the prostate crowds against the rectum, with the bladder above, and is surrounded by the sphincters that handle urinary control. The urethra runs through the middle of the prostate like Interstate 80 through Nebraska.

As if festooned with festive bunting, the prostate surface is draped with arteries and veins, plus wee gossamer nerves. Because of its tricky location, Walsh states, ". . . any form of treatment for prostate cancer can produce side effects including incontinence, impotence, and rectal bleeding."

Charming.

Walsh dives into the importance of prostate fluid in reproduction, then divides the prostate organ into zones modeled after New York City's five boroughs, complete with high taxes and a shortage of cabs. One zone is the peripheral, the very spot selected for my unpleasant biopsy. Seems that most prostate cancers—72%—develop in the peripheral zone.

Furthermore, the tissue that makes up the prostate wall is thinner than a Hollywood promise of future pay. Should cancer grow within the prostate, it can, in time, penetrate the organ's wall, also known as the capsule. Walsh says the cancer then "starts to creep along the wall of the prostate, heading north toward the seminal vesicles, in advanced cases ultimately extending into the bladder, the urethra, and the pelvic side walls."

Bad news.

Followed by somewhat good news.

Most prostate cancer is adenocarcinoma (95%). It produces no symptoms and is slow growing, almost governmental in its torpidity. So your best bet is to catch it early. Otherwise, if allowed to mature, "[prostate cancer] can produce terrible symptoms and excruciating pain."

Okay. Pokey cancer. Cool.

Flipping ahead, I discovered chapters with attractive titles such as: "Molecular Causes of Prostate Cancer: The Double Attack of Oxidative Damage and Inflammation." My eyes blinked like semaphore lights aboard an ancient ship. How bad was my case?

I decided to reexamine my crumpled, tear-stained biopsy report.

CHAPTER 3

WEEP, THEN READ IT

Had I paid attention back in Trachmann's office, I might've learned that my report contained crucial information regarding my cancer's aggressiveness, how far it had spread, and the odds for a successful cure. I studied the Walsh book, skipping around for the information necessary to understand my report.

First off, to draw a bead on the tumor's aggression, I needed to decipher my Gleason score. It seems prostate cancer cells are divided into five patterns based on how the cells appear under a microscope. (This in addition to the previously mentioned five boroughs.) The cell patterns are numbered 1 to 5 in order of aggression— five being most bellicose, rude, and indifferent to your life plans.

Peering through the lens, a doctor observes the cancer samples, appearing like malignant Rorschach blots, some more fragmented than others. He counts the five cell pattern types, noting which are most common. An equation is then formed. The most common is added to the second most common. The answer is your Gleason score. Walsh explains, "The lowest possible Gleason score is 1 + 1 = 2; the highest is 5 + 5 = 10."

Scores of 5 and 6 occur frequently, indicating slow growing tumors with an excellent shot at a cure. Seven is also common, but means the cancer is a tad more encroaching.

My Gleason score was 3 + 4 = 7.

Somewhat rapacious, but better than 4 + 3. Such a score would reveal that the most common cancer cells present in my prostate were also high in aggression. If one must have a seven, 3 + 4 is the preferred equation.

Next I needed to decipher the extent to which the cancer might have spread. For that, I needed to know my TNM rating. TNM Classification of Malignant Tumors system breaks down like this: "T" represents the local extent of the tumor; "N" indicates metastases to the lymph nodes; "M" indicates distant metastases, or, sadly, Mr. Cancer has flown off on a wild ride.

My stage description was T1c.

While only a prediction, less is more in the TNM world. T1s are way cool, indicating there's little chance the cancer has escaped the prostate. On the pathology report, my urologist broke down T1c yet further. He'd scribbled that I stood a 63% chance of the cancer still being confined to my prostate. Nevertheless, a 30% chance existed that the cancer might've migrated outside the capsule. As for the tumor reaching the nearby seminal vesicles (a pair of glands that pass fluids into the ejaculatory duct) those odds rolled in at a weak 6%. Could the cancer have spread to my lymph nodes? According to the data, there was no more than a 2% shot.

Like a fat man on the bus, expansive cancer always looks for more room to set down its Big Gulp. Because nerve cells are usually surrounded by empty space (and many nerves lounge about the prostate's surface like day workers outside a lumber yard), my biopsy also checked for something called perineural invasion. Though distressing, this is not a game-changer as such escaping cancers may still be cured.

On my report, I lacked an identifiable perineural invasion.

So my Gleason score and TMN indicated I'd acquired a slightly aggressive cancer, but the odds favored it remaining inside the prostate. What were my chances for a successful cure?

To answer that, I checked my Gleason score (7), PSA (6.3) and clinical stage (T1c) against the Partin Tables. Walsh compares the tables to "virtual surgery—they help predict what would be found if the prostate were removed surgically and examined by a pathologist. [Partin Tables] provide an excellent way to predict the chances of a cure—the odds that local treatment will eliminate the disease forever and that no cancer cells have escaped the prostate."

Of course, Walsh and Partin invented the tables in the first place, but they're based on the results of thousands of surgeries at Johns Hopkins. The tables are statistics. As I was learning, statistics aren't the final word. But you've got to base your decisions on something. Besides, I liked the data coming out of the Partin Tables—and Han Tables. (Cancer statistics have more tables than Caesar's Palace.)

Scrawled across my report like a spelling test grade, Trachmann had written 81%. That meant an 81% chance of a successful operation with clear surgical margins—no cancer cells outside the prostate. As mentioned, prostate cancer is multifocal, sprouting like kudzu—five of my 12 samples showed tumors—you couldn't pluck off those tumors like nettles from a trouser leg. The safest course was to remove the whole prostate, then go out for tacos and beer. (Except the patients; most of them return home in one or two days.)

Matters could be worse. For example, Team in Training is a fund-raising group whose participants raise money to battle blood cancers while training for various distance events. Having been an assistant marathon coach with a local team, I'd learned more than I cared to about aggressive carcinomas such as leukemia, lymphoma, Hodgkin's and non-Hodgkin's lymphoma, and multiple myeloma. These were fast, ruthless cancers.

From diagnosis to Forest Lawn Memorial Park might only take months.

Joy and I liked the 81% odds.

Now what?

CHAPTER 4

CANCER COUNTRY

█ 'd undergone two major and one minor surgery over the last five years. The thought of another operation depressed me. But my choices were limited. Further Walsh readings indicated a trio of treatment options:

A. Active surveillance;

B. Surgery;

C. Radiation.

I recalled a blood test once that revealed a surge in my bilirubin—something in the liver. My doctor was concerned and recommended a specialist. I never went, did nothing, changed nothing. Within a year, the bilirubin returned to normal levels and stayed there. So what if my prostate cancer held steady, content with its current station, lacking the malicious ambition of blood cancers?

In the world of prostate cancer, such an approach is called active surveillance. Similar to what the NSA does to American citizens, active surveillance involves monitoring. Unlike the NSA, it only monitors changes in the PSA level and not the phone calls of reporters or ex-girlfriends. With my health care evaporating in 50 days, active surveillance might be perfect, only involving bi-annual office visits and a pair of blood tests.

Sadly, prostate cancer wasn't bilirubin. Once mutations marred my DNA, (oxidative damage), I had prostate cancer . . . period. In addition, because of my relatively youthful age (61), Walsh felt active surveillance was not an indicated treatment.

That left radiation and surgery.

Surgery suited men "fit to undergo the procedure without an increased risk of complications, and who are going to live long enough to need to be cured." (My dearest wish.) Back in the day, prostate cancer surgery wasn't for the faint-hearted. A grisly procedure: patients were sliced open like blue gills, from pubic bone to naval. With the incision held open with C-clamps, doctors carved around in a lake of blood, hoping they sundered the right parts. Afterwards, you were impotent, with a 25% chance of incontinence, wondering what in the name of hickory just happened.

Such a procedure is called retropubic surgery. Of course, today's operating techniques and equipment are vastly improved. In fact, my friend Harry was recently diagnosed with prostate cancer and selected retropubic surgery. On Facebook, he posted a photo of his whopping big scar. Why did he choose this method? I can't say. I think he had a discount from Groupon.

Nowadays, the hot surgery is robotic radical prostatectomy, far less invasive than retropubic. Across your abdomen, the surgeon makes a number of small incisions like lane dividers. Then, sitting at a computer screen, and using robot hands and a flashlight, he would enter through the small incisions and remove the prostate.

Are there drawbacks? I read about one in *The Weekly World News*. Several years ago in Tokyo, four robot prostatectomy devices activated on their own. Late at night, they crept from the hospital and assaulted men in the Ginza, removing their prostates regardless of condition, need, or ability to pay. Afterwards, the devices returned quietly to the hospital before dawn. No one knows why. What are you going to do? It's Japan. They marry their sex robots.

Which brings us to radiation.

Radiation would be a commitment to a process. Walsh says that a major advantage to surgery "is that it gives some early, definitive answers. In contrast, when men undergo radiation therapy, there is no pathologic specimen to evaluate, and many patients find this unnerving." But perhaps the incontinence and impotence risks weren't as severe?

For prostate cancer there are two major kinds of radiation: external-beam and brachytherapy. External beam involves radiation beamed into the tumors from outside the body. As for brachytherapy, it implants radioactive seeds directly into the tumor. Both methods are very high-tech, very precise, and depend on your Gleason score, PSA, Partin Tables, etc. As it turned out, I was not a candidate for brachytherapy. This didn't bother me. After the biopsy, I didn't want anything up my butt, especially radioactive seeds.

From what I'd read in Walsh, incontinence and impotence factors are present with radiation, but arrive over time. There's also fatigue and increased bowel movements.

Since cancer is a family disease, my wife and mother-in-law were also reading Dr. Walsh's book. Radiation seemed okay, but a consensus was forming in our little family, leaning toward the one-stop shopping of surgery.

In mid-August, I met Trachmann again. Wearing a parrot-print shirt, he looked fresh and rested from his South American holiday. Once more, Teal Scrubs acted as court reporter. Recently, I found a sheet of yellow legal paper with my medical questions written down in pencil. Here's one: "Why is there less bleeding in a radical retropubic prostatectomy if the patient gets spinal or epidural anesthesia?" Such boring bullshit was clearly designed to make me look clever. But I did have a few pertinent inquiries:

Me: "Is there a window after which the 81% successful surgery odds decline?"

Trachmann: "Today, your cancer is at a manageable stage. But it's too advanced for watching. If we hold off another few months there's every possibility the tumors will grow and penetrate the capsule, possibly spread to the seminal vesicles, lymph nodes, or even the bloodstream. Then treatment becomes more complicated."

Teal Scrubs: (Soft keyboard tapping.)

Me: "You know my union health care runs out on September 30th."

Trachmann: "We can slide things around; schedule you for surgery before the end of next month. Or you can begin radiology. But first get a second opinion. Then decide on a form of treatment. I'd recommend meeting with a radiologist in case you choose that direction. But you'll need to move now on all this."

Teal Scrubs: (Soft keyboard tapping.) "This laptop is hot."

CHAPTER 5

RADICAL THOUGHTS

A few people I knew worked locally in medicine. I asked around. Trachmann's reputation was good. Prostate surgery was his bread and butter, meat and potatoes, kale and bean sprouts. He operated every week at a hospital equipped for, and familiar with, radical prostatectomy. He also seemed to do quite well at restoring his patients' continence and sexual abilities.

Still, I made an appointment with another urologist.

A week later, in a small crowded office, I met with Urologist #2, Dr. Albertson, a tall, pale man, perhaps 70 years old. Examining the biopsy report, Albertson mulled over my Gleason score, PSA, and TNM. Conclusion: were he my age, he'd probably opt for surgery. As we were wrapping things up, he asked about my past surgeries. I mentioned an operation I'd undergone while in the service on Okinawa. Turns out Albertson had been a young army doctor, once stationed in the same hospital that treated me.

Me: "Camp Kue? No kidding?" (Pronounced 'Coo-wee.')"

Albertson: "1970 to '71. We still treated a lot of 'Nam casualties."

Me: "I was at Kue in '72. My ward got in Marine advisors, wounded at Quang Tri City."

Albertson: "I haven't heard anyone say 'Kue' in over forty years."

Me: "We smoked on the ward, watched movies, and every night they gave us outstanding drugs."

Albertson: "Quite a time."

Me: "Oh, yeah."

By now it was the last few days of August. Following Trachmann's advice, I met with the radiation doctor. Fairly young, early 40s, Radiation Doc showed me around his TomoTherapy Hi-Art System. He walked me through the procedures, the MRIs, the Intensity Modulated Radiation Therapy, three-dimensional images, the side effects. Because wriggling patients threw off the radiation beams, the clinic made a body mold to help keep patients absolutely still. I learned I might experience rectal bleeding. RD also confirmed that my Gleason score rendered me a poor candidate for radioactive seeds. I brushed back a tear.

Back home, Joy and I reviewed our status: medical, health insurance, financial. Time was short. We needed to choose a procedure, book a start date for either surgery or radiation, then line up new health insurance. Talking it over, we officially discarded radiation, especially since treatment would overlap with the new insurance—which might not include Radiation Doc. Surgery it would be. Our finances still sucked, but I raided my 401k, plus my mother-in-law floated us a loan that would help carry Joy and me through the next two months.

Right after Labor Day, I met Trachmann.

Me: "Mark me down for a radical prostatectomy."

Trachmann: "I'll slot you in before the end of the month. You'll have the operation and probably be home the next day."

Of course, this was before I learned about the Bell Curve.

Two days later, one of Trachmann's Paperwork Gals called. There'd been a cancellation. Monday, September 22 was open. Would that day be acceptable for a radical robotic prostatectomy? Sure. After she hung up I gulped: no more theory; the bullet was in the chamber.

With a date locked in, my wife began searching for our next health care provider. With a 40% chance of reacquiring skin cancer, I required bi-annual dermatology checkups. But during that time, we were obsessed with prostate surgery. (That focus would cost me later.) Our new insurance must cover Trachmann.

Busy and stressful, the next few weeks zipped by. My sister visited from Seattle, offering her support. I returned to my primary care physician for a pre-op physical, blood work, EKG, chest x-ray (bilirubin normal). A death in the family required a trip north to San Francisco. And a procedure needed to be in place for notifying friends and family about my upcoming operation. Not wishing to be another cancer victim on social media, I assembled a list of people that Joy could email with updates.

Now a week out from the operation, I was required to donate blood. (Interesting fact: God the Good Hospital validated parking for blood donors, but not surgical patients.) According to Walsh, less than one percent of robotic prostatectomy patients needed a blood transfusion. Hence the hospital would probably return my blood in an old Gatorade jar with a celery stalk. After the procedure, I received ferrous sulfide pills to be taken three times a day at meals. These iron pills turned my poo black. Everything I expelled looked like Satan's dung.

Lovely.

CHAPTER 6

STUFFED

Four days out from surgery, I returned to the hospital for an extensive medical debrief. A nurse keenly noted all my old diseases and illnesses with an emphasis on previous operations. I mentioned the appendectomy scar on my abdomen, assorted wounds to thigh and calf, knee surgery—too many marathons—basal squamous cancer surgery involving skin grafts to my snout. (Fortunately the graft took, or I would have ended life looking like a star-nosed mole.) Shoulder surgery to sand down a bone spur. There's no rebate on the human body and I'd wrung fair use out of mine.

On Friday, September 20, Joy and her mom treated me to an Italian dinner at a nice restaurant. (I wouldn't eat a full meal again for some time.) Weekend nutrition would consist of pills, laxatives, antibiotics, magnesium citrate, then nothing including water after midnight on Sunday.

Over the weekend, munching popsicles, I checked in again with Walsh. What exactly would happen to me Monday? Not pretty. My stomach and pubic area would be shaved; a breathing tube shoved down my mouth to the lungs; I'd be pumped full of gas, then tilted practically upside down; eyes packed in Vaseline to keep them moist during the three and a half-hour procedure. Then robot arms would cut out my prostate. If Earthmen were kidnapped by an alien race and treated that way, there would be a savage war in space until every alien molecule pulsed a cold, radioactive blue.

("I know a guy whose cousin was there. He told me the whole thing."

"No shit."

"Pumped 'em full of gas, then packed their eyes in friggin' Vaseline."

"Son-of-a-bitch."

"Then these 'bots ripped out everybody's prostate. They use 'em for kids' toys."

"Alien filth. We oughta fix their asses."

"Don't worry. We fried 'em all with space napalm.")

Pithy dialogue aside, there were ergonomic reasons in play. As said, the robotic prostatectomy surgeon— Trachmann—would have to work in a tiny space amongst bladder, rectum, sphincter and nerve bundles that control erections. To create elbowroom, the medical team would pump in carbon dioxide and bloat my abdomen, spreading out the organs. There is even a medical term for this, insufflation—the act of blowing something into a body cavity. (Say the word. Roll it around. Whisper "insufflate" as if to a lover.) Then the bottom of the operating table would be elevated so my big feet rose above my head. This would cause my intestines to shift into the upper abdomen, giving Trachmann yet more working space for his fine robot arms. Next, sharp little surgical instruments, looking like a pencil with dagger handles, would be placed in my abdomen through small incisions (very close to my old appendix scar). Called trocars, these dagger handles act like Starbucks splash sticks. When the surgeon's ready to insert a robot arm or a ray of some kind, out come the trocars.

Walsh continues: ". . . surgeons make an incision just above the rectum. The prostate is gradually separated from the rectum, bladder, urethra, and vas deferens [sperm transport ducts]. The seminal vesicles are removed along with the prostate, and then the bladder is linked once again with the urethra."

I can study aircraft reports and pilot profiles all I like. But if I want to fly to Chicago, I'll need to trust the pilot. Having researched, I knew Trachmann cut his surgical teeth on old-school, carve-'em-up-the-belly stuff. If the high-tech robotic prostatectomy computer screen flashed a 401 Error, I was confidant Trachmann could carry on. He wouldn't need someone holding up a smart phone set to WebMD.

That weekend, I fretted: would Trachmann slice out all the cancer? Would he rebuild my urethra, connecting it to the bladder so I didn't spend the rest of my life as Captain Leaky? And would he spare the appropriate number of neurovascular bundles so that I could still have an erection, not drifting through my Golden Years as flaccid and impotent as the U.S. Congress?

Sunday night I said my prayers and slept well. I'd done all I could to prepare. Tomorrow, they'd wheel me in and knock me out. I'd awake minus a cancerous prostate, and be back home Tuesday.

Or so I'd been told.

CHAPTER 7

WE CONTROL YOU

On the morning of the operation, I packed light. Sleep apnea being one of my numerous maladies, I grabbed my CPAP machine, a sleep mask, a book, a toothbrush, and a change of underwear. What else would I need? After all the pressure and running around and medical blah blah since August, I was eager to see the operation in life's rearview mirror. All the tension had been rough on Joy. With me in the hospital, she could finally nab some rest.

Only a fifteen-minute drive from our house, God the Good Hospital welcomed me that sunny morning with additional paperwork. Ah, but all was not one-sided. The hospital provided us with a thick booklet informing Joy and me how committed they were to my safety and comfort. They pledged to provide excellent care during my stay. And they would ask if I had pain—mostly I would tell them—and help manage it.

("Take deep breaths.")

Escorted to pre-op, Joy and I found ourselves in the surgical on-deck circle. There I changed once more into a fashionable back-less gown, then climbed into a wheeled bed. Wearing sweaters and pastel scrubs in the chilly air, friendly nurses stopped by, asking my name and date of birth as they affixed plastic wrist bands with my name and date of birth plus a barcode containing my name and date of birth. Joy gathered up my clothes, wristwatch, and CPAP machine, then we waited and smiled back at the nurses.

As I understood things, I would be the leadoff operation at 12:30 PM. Hopefully, Trachmann would wrap around 3:30 or 4:00 PM, meaning I'd awaken in post-op, say between 4:30 and 5:00 PM. Once I was conscious, the hospital would probably park me in intensive care. Joy and I figured she should split then, while I slept off the drugs.

Having brought her laptop, Joy checked various online health care matters while I started a book by Jerzy Kosinski called *The Painted Bird*. Either a somewhat autobiographical—or completely fictitious—account of the author's childhood in Eastern Europe during World War II (opinions vary), the narrative described scenes of pitiless, unmerciful cruelty. I stopped reading and smiled at the nurses.

A young nurse arrived, interested in opening an IV line in my arm. That way the medical staff could insert drugs, fluids, Red Bull, etc. Selecting a nice bluish vein in my right hand, she jabbed in a needle, shoved, shoved harder, apologized, then withdrew the needle. A second attempt also ended in defeat.

My hand hurt and I said so. Choosing a fresh vein, she jabbed-shoved-apologized-withdrew. Fortunately, the nurse recognized facial cues indicating angry impatience. Apologizing, she called over a middle-aged co-worker with sandy hair and round glasses. Clearly a pre-op veteran, Sandy Hair sunk needle into vein on the first go.

My anesthesiologist dropped by. I recalled Kue Hospital, pre-op morphine and a dreamy blissful state. I asked what she'd be using on me. Peeved, the woman rattled off a list of drugs as if she'd been sued for the information. ("Outrageous! A patient curious about what entered his body! Such cheek!") She disappeared into a gathering crowd of friendly men and woman—the Scrub People—who asked my name and birthdate, administered drugs, transferred me to a gurney and attached IV and tubing, then wheeled me out of pre-op. Joy and I waved "bye."

Pushing the gurney was a young upbeat guy sporting a very large, blue paper hat. The hat looked like something worn by a pizza chef. We turned here. We turned there. We rolled down a long corridor toward stainless steel double doors, then boom! Surgical Land. All the locals wore pizza chef hats. My guy was slick. Without slowing the gurney, he snatched up a pizza chef hat, setting it on my head so I blended.

Whatever drugs I'd been given were starting to kick in. (It wasn't morphine, but so few things are.) Into the operating room we rolled. I could see a white erase board, a list of names, but not mine. One-two-three and I was transferred to another, narrower gurney. Rather nippy in the OR. (Temperatures are lowered to reduce infection risk.) Bustling about were OR nurses, surgical techs, physicians' assistants, and residents, one of whom had smuggled in a package of crackers and was being chided by superiors.

A male voice from behind and above addressed me in a steady, reassuring tone. Another injection was administered.

Long ago, they knocked you out with gas. Creepy. (Afterward, you puked like a sick cat.)

First, a rubber mask would be fitted over nose and mouth. Next, a medical authority figure would say, "Count out loud backward from a hundred." I made it down to 97 when my field of vision dissolved into blackness filled—literally—with the letter "Z" in different fonts and sizes, speeding toward me in a wild parallax effect. A few seconds, then buh-bye. *Poof!*

One moment you're conscious, the next moment you're conscious somewhere else, but time has passed. It's like being a blackout drinker.

This time, the most recent injection must've been the "good-night" drug. I remember thinking my new gurney felt confining. Would Trachmann and his robotic arms have space to work?

Poof!

CHAPTER 8

MAN WITHOUT A PROSTATE

Bright lights; an indistinct face loomed above me.

A female voice announced to someone that I was awake. Minus my glasses, everything was blurry as faces darted around my peripheral vision. My throat felt horrible, scraped raw as if I'd spent several hours with a dirty tent pole jammed down my windpipe. Oxygen tubes filled both nostrils, while all around me, medical devices beeped, clicked, whirred. Faces checked my vital signs. Speaking in a raspy whisper, like an actor hamming up a death scene, I croaked, "What time is it?"

The female voice answered, "A little after 8:00 PM. This is intensive care. Once you stabilize, you'll be moved to the surgical ward."

So late. What happened? Was my operation delayed? Had I been parked in frosty Surgical Land with my feet in the air? Queued up behind other gurneys like a Honda Civic at Jiffy Lube?

Where was Joy?

Sensations returned with all the speed of geological time. Bloated by gas, my stomach ached as if I'd swallowed a child's inflatable swimming pool. Little position shifts set off a rattling and clacking of tubes, lines, and sundry medical attachments. Many of these attachments were connected to a stainless-steel pole, perhaps six-feet tall. Any restless thrashing made me sound like a fully decorated Christmas tree sneaking out of the house.

Still drug-woozy, I found myself underway once more. Wheeled out of intensive care, I was rolled into another stainless steel-sided elevator. Up we rose to the Surgical Ward; past a long desk manned by a woman in scrubs, face plastered to a computer screen, along a well-lit corridor smelling very disinfected, into a dark, single-patient room.

Overhead light illuminated the bed from above and behind. Across the room, I saw a silent TV attached to the wall. I heard my wife—*huzzah!*—talking to the Faces, something about my CPAP machine. The Faces wouldn't allow me its use until a technician checked it out. Of course, I was still hooked up to oxygen. My apnea manifested as shallow or paused breathing, and I required flowing air to sleep. Nevertheless, an absence of sleep would become one of several sore points, as medical matters slid sideways.

Joy and I finally made eye contact. Later, she told me I looked ghastly: distressed, in pain, and exceptionally pale—since I'm Irish, that's really saying something. Along with the aching throat, a sharp pain began welling up around my bladder. Joy mentioned speaking to Trachmann around 6:00 PM. I guess my surgery was tougher than expected thanks to resistance from the scar tissue around my old appendix incision. Still, Trachmann had deemed the procedure a success, prostate out, and no evidence of spreading cancer—"negative margins" being the medical phrase. Exhausted, Trachmann split. Joy blasted out an email update to our family-friends list, then set off on a husband quest, searching this room and that wing, asking a nurse, then some lad in scrubs, finally locating me on the 7th floor.

Physical discomfort hollowed out the triumph. Feeling as if a bowie knife were jabbing my abdomen, I couldn't appreciate the possibility of being prostate cancer free. Instead, I croaked for a pain pill. Joy relayed the information to a Face, busy taking my vitals. At this point, I should describe the six-foot stainless-steel pole that I came to call the Click-Whirr.

With a star-shaped base and five wheels, the Click-Whirr held my IV drip, with hooks for additional medical bags. In addition, a box-like electronic device regulated the amount of fluids my body received from such bags, making a click-whirr sound every eight seconds.

(As an experiment, set your smart phone timer to eight seconds. Then retire for the evening. Whenever the timer beeps, say "click-whirr." Meanwhile, attempt to sleep.)

Should the hanging bags of saline, plasma, antibiotics, and Red Bull run low, the Click-Whirr emitted a double warning beep, followed by ten seconds of silence, then another double beep. This beepbeep-quiet-beepbeep sequence continued until manually muted. (Eventually, I located the mute button. But that night, I required a nurse to silence the rotten thing.) However, no sooner would my machine shut up, then double beeps sounded outside the room from other Click-Whirrs in other rooms across the ward, crying out like strange nightbirds seeking a mate.

Hooked to my bed were a catheter and a drain. The Foley Catheter was a thin tube inserted into my penis and funneling urine into a big plastic bag. It was named after some Irish guy who originally emptied them for whiskey money. In addition, there was the plastic Jackson-Pratt drain. About the size and shape of a hand grenade, the bulb collected wound fluids via plastic tubing stitched to one of my incisions.

Noisy Click-Whirr had many control lights. If not turned to the wall, Click-Whirr's lights bounced off a mirror above a small sink beneath the television and reflected back onto the bed. More light emanated from the nurse's computer, plus assorted other medical devices around the room. Corridor brightness spilled under and around a curtain near the door. With the staff popping in frequently to check my vitals, the room door tended to stay half open.

Seeing I was exhausted and annoyed, Joy kept trying to silence the Click-Whirr. At last, my first pain pill arrived. The pill was called Norco. This is either a brand name, or a desert city in Riverside County where the drug is manufactured in bulk. Whatever the case, it provided fast relief. Pain blocked, I told Joy to take off. Even in my dopey state, I knew she was done in after a long anxious day. A hospital tech checked out my CPAP machine. It wouldn't work. Great. But I still had oxygen in the nose and my eye mask to eliminate ambient light. For a time, I dozed off.

Click-whirr. . . . . click-whirr. Beep-beep . . . . beep-beep.

Along with checking my vitals, staff buzzed around me, emptying the Jackson-Pratt drain and refreshing my antibiotics. After a few hours, pain flared and I craved again the company of Good Sir Norco.

I tossed and turned.

CHAPTER 9

TUESDAY BLOODY TUESDAY

Drugged up and weary, I removed my sleep mask, slick with surgical Vaseline from around my eyes. Grayish light slowly filled the room like old age. Carts rattled outside in the corridor; a loudspeaker paged Dr. Hebert to report to orthopedics. Glancing about, I noticed a dresser near the bed with an old-fashioned princess phone. (Did the hospital sub-lease this room to teenage girls from the 70s?) A window to my left opened up on a small park below. On the wall across from the bed, a dry erase board featured the names of the charge nurse, RN, and assistant nurse. (Each RN serviced five patients, so no one got stuck with all the needy cases like me.) In addition to the nurse's computer station, the aforementioned small sink and TV, there was a crucifix mounted above the door, possibly for emergencies when the nurse call button failed. In the corner furthest from the door stood an odd, hexagonal-shaped bathroom/shower with a frosted glass door. It reminded me of the teleportation chamber in *The Fly*.

I wasn't alone.

Wearing a white doctor's coat, Trachmann stood at the foot of the bed.

In a quiet voice, he informed me I had post-op complications.

Remember how the urethra runs through the prostate like I-80 through Nebraska? Imagine you removed Nebraska, but wanted to keep I-80 intact. You'd need to marry the interstate to Wyoming and Iowa. Matters weren't dissimilar with the prostate. The urethra was now hooked up to the bladder. The new join was called the anastomosis.

Fuzzy-headed, I listened as best I could while Trachmann explained that urine sometimes leaks from the anastomosis into the body, or a blood clot might enter it. Infection, fluid buildup, stress and pain were frequent hallmarks of the wayward anastomosis. More tests would be required.

I would not be going home today.

In the meantime, the nurse entered the room. Trachmann asked if she'd walked me around last night. Upon hearing "no," doctor invited the nurse into the corridor and delivered a crisp lecture. ("When I say I want him walked it's an order, not an option.")

Walsh mentions something called the "clotting cascade—a chain of events that cause the blood to coagulate." While this cascade can halt bleeding during traumatic events, it can be bad news post-surgery. Should a blood clot form in the legs' deep veins (thrombosis), the clot can shoot straight up into the lungs and kill your sick ass. Since sluggish blood flow leads to clot formation, Trachmann was correct in wanting me walked ASAP.

However, I had been an inert physical wreck ten hours earlier, and I wasn't much better now. Lobster-sized scorpions scuttling up the sheets wouldn't have gotten me up, let alone out a'walking. After Trachmann split, I told the nurse, "Sorry you got reamed, but leaving me alone was the right call."

She smiled, "Oh, thanks. That happens sometimes."

She said they might try draining the anastomosis region and relieving pressure. This would allow the leak—if leak it was—to heal. I sure as hell didn't want another operation.

With a rattle of trays, breakfast arrived. I sampled a bit of Jell-O and a little coffee. Everything tasted like bile, even a sip of water. A nurse suggested the taste could be from the surgical gas. Still as bloated as an exercise ball, I pushed the tray away.

Joy arrived later that morning, just in time to help the nurse sit me up for a walk. My Click-Whirr needed to be detached from the wall and set to "battery." My Jackson-

Pratt drain was pinned to the second hospital gown I wore, the one that covered my unsightly butt. Transferring the catheter bag from the bed to the Click-Whirr, the nurse examined the contents. She turned to my wife.

"He's not draining very much."

Was this intimate knowledge women shared? How full a catheter bag should be on any given day? Like colors that clashed?

A gaggle of wife, nurse, and Click-Whirr surrounded me as I shuffled out into the corridor. Staff computer stations lined one wall, each with an office chair. After around four yards, I was panting like I'd summited Everest. Angling for the nearest computer station, I collapsed into the chair. Eventually, my gaggle got me back into bed.

Since last night, I'd grown paler; my face was now whiter than a country club on Martha's Vineyard. Concerned, the nurse checked vitals. My blood pressure was falling. Within the hour, the very blood unit I'd donated the previous week now hung from the Click-Whirr. After the staff removed my untouched lunch, an assistant nurse stopped by and remarked to me that my catheter wasn't very full. I had no opinion, but was glad to be included in the conversation.

Still battling the stabbing pain in my abdomen, I was eager for the regular Norco deliveries. They left me sleepy and dopey—five dwarfs shy of a Disney movie.

Joy sat on a small couch near the window, working laptop and phone, still trying to lock down our new insurance. That afternoon, a good friend, Chris, dropped by. I was delighted to see someone who didn't have an opinion on my catheter bag. Fortunately, he left just as my pain pill wore off.

Shifting around like a lizard on a spit, I gulped the latest pill, craving the painless state of Norco. During the day, between walking attempts, a unit of blood, and visitors, I hadn't dozed much. My unwashed hair felt slick and greasy, like a wig dug out of a landfill. Dinner arrived and departed untouched.

Joy left shortly before the 7:30 PM shift change. (Surgical Ward nurses worked three 12-hour shifts a week and generally favored such an arrangement.) New Night Nurse checked my vitals, the Jackson-Pratt drain and the Foley, remarking, "Your catheter isn't draining very much." (Rolling my eyes would've requiring too much energy.) But New Night Nurse, 3N, was a problem solver. She thought a blood clot inside the anastomosis might be jamming the line between bladder and catheter bag. Such a blockage could also create fluid build-up inside me, resulting in pain. Receiving permission to flush out the line, 3N injected a solution into a shunt on the catheter's plastic tube. Shortly after, urine began filling the catheter bag. However, my abdominal pain remained.

A medical dynamo, 3N checked vitals again, concluding my blood pressure was still way too low. A decision was reached to top me off with two additional units of blood. Though the correct blood type, the new units had not been drawn from me personally. In such a case, protocol required my vitals be checked every half-hour. I knew from earlier that day that a unit required three to three and half hours to drain. As it was near 10:00 PM, blood transfusions would occupy most of the night.

Hey, who needed sleep? This was a hospital. I was here to get well.

Click-Whirr.

Double Beep.

Vitals checked every half hour.

Norco every few hours.

Corridor light spilled around the curtain. As my sleeping mask was basted in Vaseline, I left it off. Tonight would be catnaps.

For some reason, the pain amped up, more frequent, piercing. After I informed 3N, she gave me Norco and something quite strong at my next feeding. I was rendered fog-witted, groggy, like a teenager who'd scarfed his mom's downers.

Hours passed. Daylight arrived at some point, marking a first: 3N needed to empty my catheter bag. Clearly, she'd nailed the blockage. But then we quarreled when she wouldn't give me Norco one second sooner than the protocol indicated.

("Take deep breaths.")

Meanwhile, hanging from the Click-Whirr, the last blood unit drained. 3N was pleased, noting my blood pressure was rising. Color returned to my stubbly cheeks.

And blessed Norco returned to me.

Just then, some guy from the lab arrived.

He wanted a blood sample.

CHAPTER 10

SEPTEMBER DAZE

A black-haired doctor in green surgical scrubs stood at the foot of my bed. Dr. Tony Deckhouse was assuming Trachmann's rounds. Lacking sleep, heavily medicated, I thought I heard Deckhouse say that Trachmann was down in Texas, where every year he and several colleagues purchased plague-infested monkeys from the government, then shot them in an old corn silo. Or else Trachmann was at a medical conference. One of the two.

Deckhouse inquired after my appetite. I told him everything tasted like bile. A nurse assistant entered just then. In a thick Spanish accent, she said I had "naucha." Deckhouse tensed as if he'd warned the woman never to say "naucha" in his presence. Nevertheless, he promised to administer a drug to curb the acid reflux.

Around mid-morning, cheerful nursing students from Pierce College trooped in. Later, an RN told me the students must perform a required number of practical work hours. Made sense. She added that some students found dealing with actual patients a turn-off. These few often resigned, changing their majors to hospital administration.

Several energetic students offered to assist me on a stroll. Stumbling and weak from fatigue, I was hustled down the corridor like a drunk being rushed toward a cab. Later, I wondered how many of them quit.

An injection arrived to tame my acid reflux. At lunch, I supped upon a spoon full of Jell-O and a sip of coffee. Still the bile taste. The nurse assistant returned in the early afternoon and I was washed and shampooed. Weak and listless, I let her move me around as if I were a tranquilized dog. Afterward, I sat up in a chair and dozed. Since Sunday, I hadn't had a full night's sleep.

In the early afternoon, I received another bile-buster injection. Joy arrived and we walked around the ward. This time, I needed less help, progressing a bit further. Later, Joy made phone calls. Health care ended in six days. On the line with a representative of New Fun Health Care, Joy was preparing to seal the deal when I started puking.

Fortunately, a nurse was present. Holding a plastic, kidney-shaped dish under my chin, she caught the hurl as I threw up sips of coffee and a spoon full of Jell-O. Emptying the mess into the toilet, the nurse returned as I vomited up some rogue liquid. She caught the mess, again emptying the dish. This happened a third time, then a fourth. My performance was deemed impressive. I hadn't eaten a solid meal since Friday night and here I was barfing like a college student after finals. Maybe the injections were breaking up the stomach gas, but they seemed to be producing a naucha tsunami.

Dinner arrived, but I couldn't eat. Instead, I hiccupped. Every stich in my stomach hurt. Clearly I'd entered a new and different phase of discomfort. Progress?

Joy headed home in the early evening, taking along my Vaseline-drenched sleep mask. Distracted by puking, heaving and hiccups, I realized that the day was almost done and I hadn't summoned old chum Norco. Could breaking up that blood clot be the answer? No time to ponder, as new challenges arose.

In the world of post-op, Walsh says, "One of the most important steps in recovering from a radical prostatectomy is the recovery of the gastrointestinal tract—mainly, this means the return of normal bowel movements. This return to normal happens much faster and with fewer complications if the bowels are empty when you undergo surgery."

My intestines were empty then and positively empty after Puke Fest. Still, the staff expressed an interest in seeing the contents of my bowels. (I hope to this day it was for medical purposes.) That evening, a New Night Nurse told me, "You need to pass gas."

I can't fart on command—never could—but I promised to be mindful of her request. Not long after, I disgorged gas several times, expelling a black spray that exited with force, leaving small crap flecks sprinkled across the sheets like caraway seeds on a Kaiser Roll. Then I sat in the unpleasant mess until the nurse assistant changed the linen and helped me clean up. This happened a second time.

Later that evening, I told A3N, "If I expel gas, I spray."

"Well, then, go to the bathroom."

Brilliant. An epiphany! Of course, I'd tried that already and noticed drawbacks. First, I needed to raise the bed up since I was still too weak to stand unaided. Then I'd have to focus on blocking gas expulsion while I transferred my catheter from the bed to the Click-Whirr. Next, I'd have to unplug the Click-Whirr from the wall, letting it operate on battery power. Following that, my Jackson-Pratt plastic-hand-grenade-of-blood had to be pinned to my hospital gown.

Carefully standing, still blocking the gas, I would scuff off to the bathroom with my Click-Whirr, open the frosted glass door of the teleportation chamber, plop down on the toilet seat, and pray the gas actually expelled. A3N listened to all this impatiently. She may've felt I was malingering.

"Well, you should try anyway."

Double Beep.

Click-whirr.

Another night passed.

CHAPTER 11

CHOW QUEST

Wearing a lab coat, Dr. Deckhouse returned Thursday morning. He seemed put-off, curt, as if I'd betrayed some trust.

"Are you eating?"

"Some."

"Passing gas?"

"Trying."

He snapped, "How can you be 'trying?' You either pass gas or you don't."

"Then I mostly don't."

"Well, you need to."

Deckhouse left. Why was he so pissed? Did he even want to be here? Perhaps he wished it were Deckhouse, not Trachmann, standing with guns blazing surrounded by howling apes. For that matter, I wished I were in the Lone Star State and not hospitalized for a fourth day.

Having slept a bit the previous night, I rose, washed, and ate a little breakfast without vomiting. Going for a walk alone, I extended the distance and could now amble along with other patients and their Click-Whirrs. Sometimes we'd exchange a few words, or nod in commiseration. Other times we'd pass each another like cars on a desert highway, focusing on the road ahead.

At lunchtime, I ate the soft stuff: pudding, Jell-O, creamed corn, a bit of applesauce. Though diminished, the reflux taste remained. Also, there lingered some abdominal pain, but not enough to utter the Norco call. If I didn't have to take a drug, I wouldn't. (A far cry from my youth.)

Spending more time sitting up in my chair, I read a few books Joy had brought. Reaching the bathroom to pass gas was far easier when sitting up. However, once I was tucked into bed, forget it: There was too much labor involved in tricking out the Click-Whirr.

In the late afternoon, I had a thought.

"Could you bring me a bed pan?"

The Nurse seemed baffled, as if I'd asked for a spittoon.

"You know, old school medicine, what everyone used to get? That way I won't have to block the gas for fear of crapping the bed."

With a tone of finality, she said, "Bed pans are for bed-ridden patients who can't get up at all."

Patiently—which was my status and state—I explained once more why rising and prepping the Click-Whirr, then scuffing to the bathroom, was really gay. She seemed skeptical, but I persisted. If the medical community wanted to ogle my stool, then they ought to play ball.

After some back-and-forth, the Nurse brought me an old-fashioned stand-alone commode. Placed beside my Click-Whirr, it was perfect. Now I needed only hold the gas until I elevated the bed, swung out my legs, and dropped onto the seat. All drains and catheters could remain in place. I felt victorious.

Emboldened, I struck out to improve my environment. If the saline drip on the Click-Whirr, or any dangling bag, neared empty, I asked that it be changed, to forestall double beeps. Studying the Click-Whirr, I located the mute button. I then asked the Nurse to ensure that no blood was drawn from me prior to 6:00 AM. (Lab techs often started their rounds at 4:00 AM, particularly if a doctor asked for a patient's blood, and wanted the data for rounds.) A nurse posted a large hand-written sign on my door, warning off early-bird techs.

In the course of working with the staff to build a quieter, darker room, I heard from one nurse who thought my issues stemmed from my being a "light sleeper." Amazing. Clearly, she was like a woman living near the elevated tracks. After a while, you don't hear the train. Also, many RNs were young mothers who hadn't enjoyed a full night's sleep in years. Hence, a patient craving more than a few hours at a time might've struck them as greedy and unnatural.

Joy arrived in mid-afternoon and we walked. By now I could navigate all the way to the end of the corridor, past a statue of the Blessed Virgin, to a waiting area near the elevators. A tall glass window offered views of nearby Griffith Park and passenger jets ascending from Burbank Airport.

That night I ate dinner, probably chicken à la king, since it would be gloopy enough to go down without a struggle. Joy left early, still looking weary. Thus, I took my final walk alone, Click-Whirr and I, rattling past the Blessed Virgin—her arms extended down with palms up as if saying, "Come ye all to me," or "I'm terribly sorry, but this is the way things are around here"—past the front desk, up the far corridor, and back down to my room. Having lapped the ward, I shut my room door and retired, gorged with success.

However, my triumphs would prove ephemeral.

CHAPTER 12

TRENDING UP

On Friday morning, I felt better than I had all week. Must've gotten at least four hours of uninterrupted sleep. And while I still tasted a little acid reflux, the abdominal pain was gone. Today, standing at the foot of the bed, was a new doctor.

Elton Raffalowitz was a husky, middle-aged fellow. Brownish hair from his forearms mingled with wrist hair, giving the impression of a lab-coat-wearing Yeti. Calm, grounded, Dr. Raffalowitz did what no other doctor or nurse had yet attempted: he explained why I was still in the hospital.

Raffalowitz said, "So, you know about bell curves?"

"Yeah; shows a distribution."

"Close enough. In the fat part of the bell are the majority of radical robotic prostatectomies. They're the patients who go home after a day or two."

"Okay."

"Then there's you. You're out on the lip of the bell with anastomosis blood clots, low blood pressure, acid reflux, and vomiting issues."

"That's me."

"And you won't eat."

"I'm doing better. So you're saying I'm a statistical anomaly?"

"You're the patient bad things happen to. There aren't many, compared to all the rest who undergo the same procedure. But that's where you guys end up, out on the lip."

"The lip of the bell?"

"Right. But you're still alive, and we can work with that."

I laughed. Raffalowitz promised another injection to eliminate the last of the naucha. I washed, shaved, ate some scrambled eggs, then took another lap around the ward. Afterward, I sat up and read. I felt pretty decent for the first time in a while.

Late that afternoon, Joy arrived and brought her mother. I was pleased to see a friendly face not wearing scrubs. We visited, they left, and I lapped the ward again. In honor of my wife, who loves English mysteries, I watched one on TV, then parked the Click-Whirr for the night. Some reflux, but my stomach seemed to be decreasing in girth. A good day.

Raffalowitz returned on Saturday morning, really pushing chow. Eat, evacuate a healthy stool, go home. Another injection for the reflux. I ate more breakfast, more lunch, took morning and afternoon laps around the ward. Spending so much time out in the corridor, I listened to the loudspeaker. Going only by names, one could assume God the Good Hospital was staffed exclusively by Jewish doctors, and run by Filipino nurses.

Early evening, and Joy walked in as I watched a college football game. As if at home, I muted the sound and watched the contest from the corner of my eye. All health news trended upward for once: shrinking stomach, no abdominal pain; stools acceptable to the medical set; a little acid reflux, but nothing meal-inhibiting. I felt less depressed and more rested, and I walked farther. Dinner rattled in and I scarfed up most of the tray. Joy split as Click-Whirr and I lapped the ward once more before retiring.

Come Sunday morning, no doctor stood at the foot of my bed. Ah, well — that's why there were golf courses. As I had on Friday and Saturday, I washed, walked, ate my breakfast, sat up and read. A nurse emptied out my full catheter and noticed the fluid in my Jackson-Pratt seemed much lighter. Assuming that was a positive, I thanked her. At lunch, I nibbled a hamburger and watched *Ghostbusters II* on TV.

Raffalowitz strolled in and said, "How'd you like to go home today?"

Well, matters suddenly grew cheerfully busy. I called Joy for a pick-up as a nurse schooled me on various medical tasks I'd need to do for myself, such as swapping catheter bags. For travel, I exchanged the hefty party-sized bag of the last week for a smaller bag that attached with elastic straps to my upper thigh. (Invisible, as long as you wore baggy sweatpants.)

As for the Jackson-Pratt, that would remain safety-pinned to my clothes for a while longer. Oh, joyous day. All week I'd dealt with immediate woes and hadn't given the future much thought—similar to high school graduation. Giddy at leaving the hospital, I was unaware that fallout from the operation was about to engulf me.

A short Mexican woman with a graying-brown ponytail arrived pushing a wheelchair. Down the corridor for the last time, past the Blessed Virgin, and to the elevators. Waiting for a car, we glanced out the window, watching a jet rise. My Wheelchair Operator wished aloud that she were onboard that faraway aircraft, bound for Las Vegas. On the elevator ride down, we talked gambling and traffic on the I-15. The woman said she used to stay at the Jade Inn. I'd always preferred a room at the mobbed-up Howard Hughes hideaway, Desert Inn.

(Gone now, and I hadn't been gaming in 14 years since I left Warner Brothers and a fat steady paycheck.)

On a bright early autumn afternoon, we waited outside the hospital. As Joy rolled up and helped me into the front seat, the woman and I did the Vegas clap, followed by palms extended outward, wishing each other "good luck."

In my case, I'd need it.

CHAPTER 13

A THOUSAND POINTS OF URINE

Wearing my baggy sweatpants, a fat warm bag of piss on my left thigh, I sat in the driver's seat of Joy's PT Cruiser. Window open, I basked in the growl of street traffic, observing the rage of Armenians engaged in a horn-honking duel in the drugstore parking lot. Meanwhile, my wife bought out the incontinence aisle. Returning to the car, I observed she'd loaded up on surgical mats, a banana-shaped hand urinal, a rectangular plastic dishpan, man diapers (in fall colors), and several sizes of antiseptic wipes. Back home, Joy placed surgical mats on the bed, my reclining chair in the living room, and on the kitchen counter in case something unexpected happened. Rummaging around, she discovered an old plastic chair so I could shower with my various attachments on. I can't recall what I watched that night on TV. I was home and happy.

But with freedom comes responsibility, such as emptying the Jackson-Pratt drain. Stitched into one of my incisions and covered by a dressing, the J-P tubing removed fluids from my wound. Employing gentle suction, this draining prevented the formation of hematomas or abscesses. Proper drain care suggested I empty J-P when the 100-milliliter container was half full, thereby avoiding back flow that could cause infection. In addition to squeezing the bulb flat to force out all the air, I'd been asked by a medical authority to record the amount, color and consistency of my drainage on a four-column form. (The last column was for comments.)

Bedtime. I swapped out the travel catheter for the party bag. No more Click-Whirr to vex me. But all was not rosy. We didn't own a hospital bed. Because staples still closed my half-dozen little stomach incisions, I could only sleep sitting up or lying on my back. Without oxygen tubes in my nose, I kept waking up for lack of air. (My new CPAP wouldn't arrive until the next day.) Plus, the pesky J-P drain seemed to always need emptying. I'd push myself to the edge of the bed, roll up, then weave down the hallway to the bathroom. First, I'd empty the party catheter into the commode. Next I'd attempt recording the amount of drain fluid. Here's my chart from Sunday evening to Monday morning:

5:00 PM   50 (mL)

9:00 PM   50 (mL) med. color

11:30 PM   40 (mL) med. color

3:45 AM   50+ (mL) med. color
                Didn't squeeze out all air – bulb popped back. (?)

8:30 AM   100 (mL) I'm very tired.

11:00 AM   40 (mL) This is stupid.

Another night of faux rest.

Because light physical activity was stressed by the medical folk, I made sure to exercise on Monday morning. Wearing baggy sweats that concealed the travel catheter and drain, I walked around the corridors of our building for ten minutes. I felt okay. An afternoon and evening lap of similar duration would be my new routine.

Back home, as I was changing clothes to shower, the doorbell rang. With Joy still sleeping, I answered wearing a towel that mostly concealed the catheter, but exposed the J-P drain, bloody tubing, dressing, the works. A young UPS guy in his mid-30s watched me sign a receipt for a new CPAP machine, eyes darting toward my medical ornaments. His facial expression said it all:

("Dear God, let me die before I end up like this human wreck.")

Monday night, Joy had a plan. We laid a surgical mat along the side of the bed, right next to my *Despicable Me* bedroom slippers. Atop the mat, Joy placed the plastic dishpan. Rather than wobble down the hall, tonight I'd sit up, empty drain and catheter into the dishpan, tote up J-

P milliliters and avoid dropping my notes into the effluvia. Come morning, I'd empty the night's slops as if it were just another day in the 18th century.

Tuesday morning we drove to Trachmann's office, a space he shared with other urologists, some of whom I hadn't yet met. Thanks to my new CPAP machine, I was semi-rested. Waiting in a small examining room, I watched as Trachmann entered solo. I asked him about his conference.

He said, "Boston. Nice city. Some of us went out for crab. Excellent."

A Band-Aid covered his right index finger.

Trachmann bore good tidings concerning my prostate biopsy. Though 20% of the organ had been cancer-ridden, no roaming adenocarcinoma appeared to have escaped. The biopsy declared the surgical margins negative. Technically, my next PSA test should read zero since nothing remained to produce Prostate Specific Antigens. I wondered if the Chinese purchased old prostates, shipping them back to the Celestial Kingdom, slicing out the cancer, mixing the rest with ginger and selling them as good luck tokens. I imagined a shop with a bell above the door, and prostates for sale, on display and clearly labeled: Political Dissident, or Christian, or Old Yankee Devil.

Scanning my J-P log, Trachmann didn't like the amount of wound drainage. Thus I'd spend another week with dear friends Jackson-Pratt and Foley. On the way down a long hall to see the Paperwork Gals, I spotted Dr. Deckhouse. He stormed past without a word, his face a mask of repressed anger as if cursing with his mouth closed. Through an office doorway, the hirsute Dr. Elton Raffalowitz talked on the phone. Wise man-yeti and I waved at one another.

Tuesday night, I terminated the J-P log. Note taking while bleary with sleep wasn't cutting it. That week, I slept better than I had for some time, but seepage continued around the drain incision. Every morning, my tee shirts would be stained with wound ooze. Continuing walks thrice a day, I gravitated outside and onto residential streets. With Jackson and Foley in tow, I kept my strolls around ten minutes. When not walking or emptying things, I attempted writing and editing a short story collection. Futile. I'd push the cursor around, rewrite the same sentence for an hour, then click over to YouTube and watch scenes from *Tropic Thunder*, or the bank shoot-out from *Heat*. No energy, no focus, not even the dogged, head-down grinding word counts that constituted most of my writing.

Around mid-week, hiccups returned, each eruption jarring my tender stomach wounds.

In the first full week of October, seven days after receiving my prostate biopsy report, Trachmann examined my stomach: still distended from the operation, but diminishing. As the color and amount of J-P fluid were deemed acceptable, Trachmann ordered the drain discontinued. Staples from my lane divider-stomach incisions were also removed. And, at last, out came the catheter. A nurse handed me a thick cotton pad to put in my underwear. Trachmann warned me that the urine was coming, as surely as a Cambodian rice farmer predicting the monsoon. Little could be done, he explained, until I underwent physical therapy. There I'd learn exercises to strengthen the underused muscles of my external sphincter.

A sphincter is a ring-like muscle constricting a body passage or orifice. As Walsh (and Trachmann) explained: "Men are equipped with three separate anatomical structures that control urine—a sphincter at the bladder neck, the prostate itself and the external sphincter (also called the striated sphincter). Radical prostatectomy knocks out two of these—the sphincter at the bladder neck and, of course, the prostate—leaving only the external sphincter to do the work of three."

That explains why a carload of guys can drive 270 miles from L.A. to Vegas in one shot, while women can't traverse forty feet of shopping mall without a pee stop. The solitary control tool I had—the striated sphincter—was the only bladder control organ women ever get. This begged disturbing questions: would I now be uncomfortable going to the restroom alone? Must we add a small couch to our bathroom? A copy of *Redbook*? Also, where did one find a striated sphincter, and what did it feel like?

Nevertheless, I was brimming with confidence. Trachmann moved on to the next patient. Cotton pad in place, I walked down the hallway to the Paperwork Gals, booking an appointment three weeks out. Leaving the office, I felt fine. The storm was past.

My wife and I stopped for breakfast. Rising an hour later after three cups of coffee, I pissed my pants as if putting out a fire in a wastebasket. Having drenched my new sporty cotton pad, I had an unpleasant feeling the storm had just returned from a short nap.

Basically, the bladder holds urine until a series of reflexes causes a bathroom urge. Bladder and sphincters then receive a message from the brain to "check flow" until an appropriate time. When you're incontinent, any time is just dandy. You can experience stress incontinence with activities that suddenly increase pressure inside the abdomen, like lifting or standing. Then there's urge incontinence, which is a sudden uncontrollable need to leak, often suffered by federal employees in Washington D.C. Finally, there's overflow incontinence — when you can't sense if the bladder was filling.

I had all three.

CHAPTER 14

WHO WILL STOP THE RAIN?

Back home I faced daily life minus bladder control. Movements gross and subtle, lying on my back, it didn't matter. Everything ended in a demoralizing urine surge. I really needed Trachmann's physical therapist. But our new insurance had other ideas.

While I moped around home like the Incredible Surging Man, Joy found that transitioning from Motion Picture Insurance to New Fun Health Care was far from seamless. I'd overhear her on the phone, voice rising in frustration as she'd be referred for answers to New Fun Health Care's website when the website was down. Or asking why a childless couple must pay twelve dollars a month for pediatric dentistry. (Obamacare fine print.) For five days, NFHC insisted we were on a plan we hadn't selected, then grandly announced our old insurance had been cancelled on October 1st. Oh, they were sharp as a paper cut over at New Fun Health Care.

Meanwhile, I tried packing my regular underwear with cotton pads. That idea cratered in less than a day. Not only were man diapers necessary, but they required cotton pads inside as well. (I was soaking through three pads a day, minimum.) Each morning, I'd wake up drenched, smelling like an interstate washroom.

Through sheer grit, Joy finally convinced NFHC we were, indeed, customers and had paid for a specific plan. Finally acknowledging same, NFHC then dithered over Trachmann's physical therapist, insisting she wasn't covered by our plan. As this particular therapist specialized in post-op continence, I desperately needed her skills. Trachmann's Paperwork Gals weighed in and saved the situation. They affirmed that NFHC carried the physical therapist, and offered to badger the insurance company on our behalf.

A week passed as I lived the life of the urine free spirit. Avoiding coffee or soda mattered little. No internal spigot staunched the constant flow. Smelling piss all the time was depressing, as if I were being forced to manufacture it for export. Three or more times a night, I'd awaken with man diapers soaked and pressure on my bladder. Sitting up, I'd whiz into a hand urinal, change, clean myself, then lie back down and hope for a little sleep before the next voiding.

After eleven days, Joy and the Paperwork Gals hacked through all the bureaucratic hurdles. I was free to book an appointment. Unfortunately, there were no physical therapist openings for another week.

I couldn't cope with seven more days.

But then a cancellation, a sudden opening, an opportunity to do more than marinate in pee. I drove for the first time since the operation, speeding out to the Valley, hopping out of the car, soaking myself. Dashing into the physical therapy building, I met Eva.

Tall with jet-black hair, late 30s, Eva was upbeat and confidant. We talked sports. She'd been a college high jumper before injuring her back. (She'd require surgery soon to fix a persistent issue.) In a small room, Eva instructed me to lie down on an examining couch, then hooked my perineal and abdominal muscles to a laptop via adhesive pads. For the next hour, she gave instruction in finding, then clenching and unclenching my striated sphincter in order to control urination. On the computer screen, I could monitor my efforts. A moving graph alerted me when I targeted the correct muscles. Called kegels, these clench-and-release exercises bolstered the pelvic floor muscles below the bladder.

(A brief digression: according to Walsh, while helpful to some, Eva's biofeedback method was "an expensive way for a man to learn how to start and stop his stream, and indeed, critical studies have demonstrated no great benefit to this elaborate and expensive procedure." I was one of the "some" who found biofeedback to be of great value. For example, I know a guy who underwent the same radical robotic prostatectomy. Afterward, his urologist tossed him a few sheets of paper with kegel exercises described on them and said *vaya con Dios*. No one told my friend you could overdo these exercises. While other factors may've been in play, his continence recovery turned out to be longer and messier than mine. Maybe a little biofeedback could've improved his condition quicker. True, I'm no doctor — but I am a man without a prostate.)

Eva then supplied me with homework: diagrammed daily exercises with frequency and duration. She also encouraged me to keep walking. My daily trio of strolls had become a habit. I mingled seamlessly with others on my street, drifting along the sidewalk with other hapless old people.

Psychologically, kegels were important. As stated, I lived with a constant dribble that could transform into a flood. At night I rose often, peeing into a hand urinal while fresh up from REM sleep. Eva's exercises provided me concrete specific actions. She also warned me against overtraining that could fatigue the striated sphincter, rendering it too tired to work. Such a result would lead to dire unpleasantness.

Five days later at my next physical therapy session, I obtained yet more exercises. I saw progress. For the first time, I could stand once or twice without pissing myself. Eva advised against trying to exert bladder control using my sliced-out prostate and bladder muscles. I would be like a legless man trying to kick a rat.

My latest goal: don't wait for pressure, but anticipate the "go" urge, then reach the toilet with something left in the bladder. I discovered that rising without excess pressure on the bladder required me to walk bent over like old time comic Groucho Marx. Mostly, after four steps, I surged. This new goal would take some fine-tuning.

Toward the end of October, Eva split for her surgery, leaving me with my exercises. Again, I grew morose. How long was this pee business going to continue? Joy saw improvement, but I thought she was trying to cheer me up. Right before Halloween, I met with Trachmann. He asked me about the physical therapy, "Are you noticing improvement?"

"I feel like a piss machine."

"Actually, you're doing pretty good as far as recovery. A lot of the discomfort you're feeling now will pass. Once you strengthen the striated sphincter, your bladder urges will stabilize."

Until then, buy stock in man diapers.

Trachmann wanted me back in a week to test my PSA. Finally, a test I wanted to flunk. But if my PSA didn't read "zero" I could be facing cleanup radiation and who knew what merry paths yet untrod.

Into November, Eva was still recovering from surgery. I continued the exercises, but feared I might've plateaued. One afternoon, I lunched with a friend.

Climbing out of the car in the coffee shop parking lot triggered a bad leak. (Stress incontinence.) Rushing inside to the washroom, I cleaned up, then sat down. Arising after lunch, the fire hose in my pants blasted again. Hurrying to the washroom, I pissed more. Amazing. It wasn't like I'd been slugging down coffee and Mountain Dew. Exiting the car at home prompted another gargantuan surge.

I spent the rest of the afternoon awash in urine and self-pity. All these exercises and my daily existence still rotated around pissing, cleaning up piss, and changing man diapers sodden with leakage. Joy told me the drug store Incontinence Aisle had changed its name to Bladder Control Aisle. I was surprised they hadn't named it after me.

CHAPTER 15

THE ROAD BACK

A week later, Trachmann announced that my PSA level tested zero. Yee-haw! *Look at me, I'm cancer free!* Then Eva returned and physical therapy recommenced.

She asked, "How's it been going?"

I said, "My wife got into the spirit of things and re-did our whole condo in yellow outdoor carpet."

Eva liked that.

With persistence, I sensed how to locate and activate my new bladder-control muscles. Eva suggested I aim to eliminate jug peeing and excessive bathroom visits. Using the striated sphincter, I should school the bladder, aiming for fewer—but more productive—bathroom trips. In the meantime, I discovered a cost-effective method of cutting down on cotton pads out in public. By inserting several sheets of double-ply toilet paper into my man diaper, I caught the wild leaks. Just toss and replace the tissue. It was easier than finding a stall and swapping out cotton pads.

Then, for two nights running, I only urinated once. By mid-November, I'd slept an entire night without awakening to pee. (I hadn't done that in almost two months.) In the morning, I loped ape-like to the bathroom and urinated. Just after Thanksgiving, I stopped wearing man diapers and returned to underwear, albeit with a cotton pad and toilet paper inside.

As affairs of micturition steadied, I rediscovered my focus and resumed writing. As we needed money, I took the only paying job available: cranking out marketing copy. ("Take advantage today of the awesome opportunity to earn the amazing cash you deserve, experience your wildest dreams, and say 'good-bye' to low-wage misery without any effort on your part!!!") In addition, I began writing a parody novel of a wildly popular romance book. Working on these projects, meeting deadlines, commissioning cover art for the book, all helped craft a daily routine not built around the life of a Leaky Man.

Challenges continued with New Fun Health Care. In our zeal to ensure Trachmann was covered, we'd failed to do likewise with my dermatologist. In early December, a routine visit led to a biopsy resulting in the discovery of yet another cancerous growth. Removing it involved a procedure with the sassy name of "burn and scrape." It also involved several hundred dollars if you weren't covered by insurance. My dermatologist charged me doctor's rates for procedure and lab—checking to see if the tissue sample was cancer-free at the miserable margins. Or I could start hunting down an NFHC dermatologist. (I'd do this later with fascinating, annoying results.) I was sick of cancer. I paid up.

For Christmas, Joy and I flew up to the Pacific Northwest to visit my sister. An adventurous time, with me unable to cross 40 feet of airport concourse without running into a washroom, jackknifed-over. I grew to be an expert at identifying tile patterns.

My odd "potty walk" would abide into 2015, but by March I could check flow and walk upright to the bathroom. My newly discovered striated sphincter knew the routine and exceeded expectations. I'd finally turned a corner.

As to sexual doings, for several months romance remained problematic. Wearing a big wet man diaper chilled my passion. (Though I understand in Hollywood there are people who pay thousands of dollars to spend an evening in such a state.) Walsh relates that in "the most skilled surgeon's hands, if both neurovascular bundles are preserved during a radical prostatectomy, potency should return in at least 80 percent of men in their forties and fifties and in 60 percent of men in their sixties." But there's a caveat, because by "age sixty, a man has only about 60 percent of the nerves he was born with—which means that if 20 percent of them are damaged by treatment for prostate cancer, only about 48 percent remain." So erectile dysfunction is not uncommon post-op, especially in older men.

So a few months passed, but thanks to Trachmann's precise cutting, the patience of my lovely wife, and a couple of boxes of Cialis, Joy and I once again enjoyed marital union. Not as often as before, but we managed to find the time, eventually ditching the Cialis.

As I slowly healed, my walks grew longer. I learned about a biometric method called Chi Running, which eases impact on knees. To my delight, a few times a week, often passed by dumpy women with fanny packs and sun visors, I was able to run again. Trotting around bridle paths and golf courses, I enjoyed the endorphins, recalling chilly mornings and long-ago marathons.

A half-year post op and I received a union script assignment. While only a short eleven-minute episode, it added sufficient hours to what I'd previously banked in 2014. Adieu to New Fun Health Care and "howdy again" to Motion Picture. Six months passed, but no more union work followed. As before, we returned to COBRA.

Having completed my first horror novel, I was working on another when the realization finally struck that my TV animation career was finished. Phone calls and emails for work had receded like an echo. When silence rings, you know you've retired. Eighteen months into post-op, I made the unofficial official. As I told a friend, retirement was indistinguishable from unemployment, except it paid better. Having worked sufficient union jobs since 1990, I qualified for a small annuity, plus health care, dental, and medication. When 65 pulled up to life's curb, with Medicare in the back seat, Motion Picture would become my supplemental.

We would COBRA no more.

Around the time of my retirement, Joy snagged a tech-writing job. Well-paying, with medical benefits, 401k and other perks, her salary eliminated our immediate financial woes, and we bought her a new car. At last, we could relax, hack away at credit card debt, and, in time, pay back Joy's mom and other family members who'd generously carried us through lean times.

Every six months, I visit Trachmann's office. Blood is drawn, my PSA reads zero, and Trachmann and I chat briefly about books, sports, history and, of course, *A Prairie Home Companion*. I'm often tempted to probe his whereabouts during my chaotic post-op week, but have decided to let sleeping monkeys lie.

Over the last three years, I've learned to live with a manageable amount of dribbling and leakage. Certain actions stress the bladder and exacerbate flow—such as excessive bending, reaching, stretching, or exercise such as stationary cycling. And while medical procedures exist that could tighten things up, I'm content to live a mostly dry life.

This year I had dinner with friends, including Chris, who'd visited me in the hospital. He mentioned having a biopsy. Eight out of twelve prostate samples tested positive for adenocarcinoma. Working as a film editor, Chris was covered by Motion Picture insurance. He used the same clinic as I. Not surprisingly, his urologist was Trachmann. I informed him there was no finer surgeon, when sober. (Trachmann laughed when I told him.)

Eventually, Chris chose radical robotic prostatectomy. Before and after the operation, we called and texted one another. He shared his anxiety. I shared my prostate cancer experience, strength and hope. A pretty good exchange.

Since my operation, four guys I know have undergone radical robotic prostatectomies. All left the hospital in one or two days.

But I ended up with a better story.

Sometimes that's worth the price.

The End

SOFT COVER EDITION UPDATE

Almost five years have passed since the operation. My PSA level continues to read zero. Incontinence remains at a manageable level, while sex, if infrequent, is pleasantly doable. I continue encountering more men who have undergone radical prostatectomies or radiation treatment. In a few cases, such as that of my brother-in-law, guys with high PSAs have been placed on active surveillance. Invariably, this leads to additional biopsies. I wish these men good health, but don't envy them.

Meanwhile, Joy and I bask in an improved financial state that allows us frills such as new clothes and vacations. My overall health is fine. Despite an injury last year, I continue to run a few times a week. I'm losing weight and have decided to train for one more marathon, to be tackled late in 2020. (I intend to write an excellent nonfiction book on running. My working title flows best if I complete a 26.2-mile course. Extreme, I know, but it's an outstanding title.) All the best!

— JP Mac
July 2019

RESOURCES

American Cancer Society statistics for 2019 estimate 174,650 new cases of prostate cancer, along with 31,620 deaths over the next year.

One man in nine can look forward to a prostate cancer diagnosis during his lifetime. As the second leading cause of cancer death in American men (lung cancer still rules), about one guy in 41 will die of prostate cancer. Chances are higher for African-American men.

Old dudes beware: The average age at the time of diagnosis is 66. My friend Chris was diagnosed in his mid-50s, but he's always been a troublemaker.

Here are a few spots to score more information. The web and YouTube are glutted with prostate cancer info; take advantage.

Prostate Cancer Foundation
https://www.pcf.org

MedicineNet
https://tinyurl.com/y9ksbvqq

International Prostate Cancer Foundation
https://tinyurl.com/y42my2ga

Online Prostate Cancer Support Group
https://tinyurl.com/yxnwfye4

His Prostate Cancer for Wives and Partners
https://www.hisprostatecancer.com

Prostate Cancer Diagnosis Video
https://youtu.be/e6h7BxOZuCU

Men's Health @ Vitaljake
https://vitaljake.com

Guide to Surviving Prostate Cancer by Dr. Patrick Walsh and Janet Farrar Worthington
https://tinyurl.com/y2p3zlqq

ADDENDUM AND ACKNOWLEDGEMENTS

Most conversations are condensed or exaggerated. Just about everyone—save Joy and I—are composites. However, the timeline, my condition, and the treatments are accurate. (When not drugged, I took notes.)

Once more, D.C. Richter rose to the occasion with her excellent cover art. A great sweeping salute to the beta readers, including Dan Hoffman, Ken Segall, and M.D. Sweeney. Joy McCann proved my wisdom in marrying her over 20 years ago, as she copyedited and proofread the final draft. Deft formatting was performed by Joya Beebe, and the fine back cover and spine design is the work of Brandi Doane McCann.

For checking over the manuscript, a special shout-out to physical therapist Cathy Kerman, MPT, SCS (Sports Injury Certified Specialist), PRPC (Pelvic Rehab Certified Practitioner).

Also kudos to Janet Farrar Worthington. The co-author of the Walsh book, Janet has shown herself to be generous in promoting my wee book and a tireless advocate for men's health issues. I humbly salute her.

A great giant fist bump to Dr. Russell Kurihara, The Old Cancer Catcher.

And, finally to my brother Men Without Prostates: On we go!

ABOUT THE AUTHOR

An Emmy Award-winning TV animation writer, JP Mac (as John P. McCann) has worked on shows such as *Animaniacs*, *Freakazoid!*, *Pinky and the Brain*, and *Kung Fu Panda*. Mac was a creative writing student of T.C. Boyle's at the University of Southern California. His short fiction has appeared in print and online in venues such as *The Best of Every Day Fiction Three* and *The Cthulhu Mythos Mega Pack*. Mac is currently writing a number of dark fantasy short stories, as well as Book Two of his Hallow Mass horror trilogy.

Check Mac's websites for publication dates.

JP Mac: https://jpmacauthor.com

Facebook
https://tinyurl.com/jpoqpd9

Write Enough! Blog
https://tinyurl.com/y34varsz

Goodreads
https://tinyurl.com/ky8q94o

A NOTE TO OUR READERS

This book is indie-published, so we remind you that reviews are pivotal in keeping our small business alive. If you enjoyed this softcover book, we strongly urge you to review it on Amazon.com so we can stay visible on that platform. Alternatively, we would request a review on Goodreads. Even a single sentence will help us out.

If you review this book in print or for an online website, blog, vlog, or podcast, please drop us a line so we can highlight your mention on social media.

— Joy McCann
Production Manager, Cornerstone Media
joy.w.mccann@gmail.com

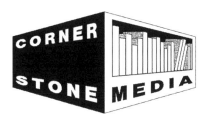

Cornerstone Media
La Cañada, California

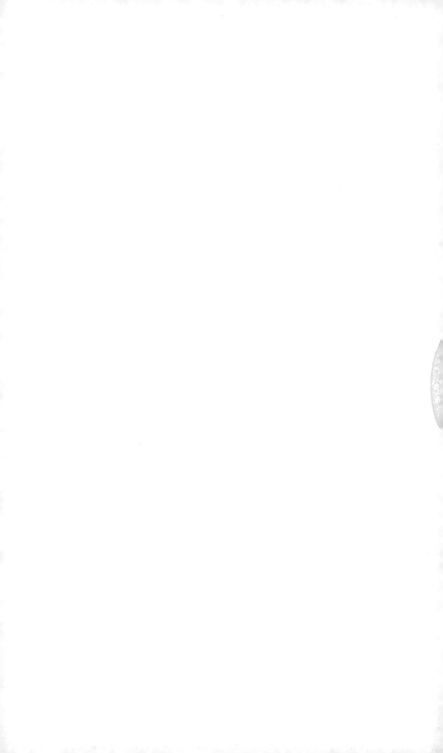

My Prostate Cancer Notes

My Prostate Cancer Notes

My Prostate Cancer Notes